NURSING HEART FAILURE SOLUTIONS

I0466533

Practical Steps for Patients Wellness

Hamish Hutton, CNS Clinical Nurse Specialist, Royal Melbourne Hospital, Australia.

Preface

Welcome to Nursing Heart Failure Solutions: Practical Steps for Patient Wellness. In the realm of healthcare, managing heart failure (HF) poses significant challenges and demands a multifaceted approach rooted in both medical expertise and compassionate nursing care. This book is a comprehensive guide designed to empower nurses and healthcare professionals with the knowledge and strategies essential for optimizing patient outcomes in HF management.

Heart failure, whether caused by structural abnormalities or intrinsic cardiac diseases, presents a complex clinical syndrome marked by compromised cardiac function. As caregivers on the frontline, nurses play a pivotal role in mitigating symptoms, promoting adherence to therapeutic regimens, and enhancing patient quality of life. From understanding the intricate pathophysiology of HF to implementing evidence-based interventions, this book equips nurses with practical tools to navigate the complexities of care. Throughout these pages, we explore the latest advancements in cardiovascular medicine, emphasizing personalized approaches to treatment and patient education. Drawing from clinical insights and research, we address the nuances of HF management, including the impact of lifestyle modifications, medication adherence, and therapeutic innovations.

This book serves as a companion for nurses dedicated to elevating standards of care in heart failure management. By embracing a holistic approach that integrates clinical expertise with empathetic patient support, we strive to empower healthcare providers in fostering resilience and wellness in their patients.

Join us on this journey as we embark on a collaborative effort to enhance the lives of those affected by heart failure, one compassionate intervention at a time.

Preface

Table of Contents

- 12.3 Reduced Anxiety Levels
- 12.4 Sound Decision-Making Regarding Care and Treatment
- 12.5 Adherence to Prescribed Self-Care Regimen

Abbreviations
- CHF: Congestive Heart Failure
- ECG: Electrocardiogram
- IV: Intravenous
- BMI: Body Mass Index
- CAD: Coronary Artery Disease
- CABG: Coronary Artery Bypass Grafting
- HF: Heart Failure
- MI: Myocardial Infarction
- BP: Blood Pressure
- HR: Heart Rate
- CVD: Cardiovascular Disease
- EF: Ejection Fraction
- ACE: Angiotensin-Converting Enzyme
- ARB: Angiotensin Receptor Blocker
- CCU: Coronary Care Unit
- ICU: Intensive Care Unit
- TTE: Transthoracic Echocardiogram
- BUN: Blood Urea Nitrogen
- CBC: Complete Blood Count
- NT-proBNP: N-terminal pro-B-type natriuretic peptide

Introduction

Heart failure (HF) stands as a formidable challenge in contemporary healthcare, characterized by the heart's inability to efficiently pump blood to meet the body's metabolic demands. This complex syndrome results from structural or functional impairments in the heart's ventricles, compromising its ability to fill with or eject blood effectively. As a progressive and chronic condition, HF necessitates comprehensive management strategies to alleviate symptoms and optimize patient outcomes.

Manifestations of HF manifest through a spectrum of clinical signs and symptoms, including fluid overload leading to pulmonary and systemic congestion, reduced exercise tolerance, and inadequate tissue perfusion. These symptoms often present as dyspnea, fatigue, edema, and exercise intolerance, significantly impacting patients' quality of life.

Understanding the diverse etiologies of HF—from chronic

hypertension and coronary artery disease to valvular abnormalities—is crucial for tailoring effective treatment plans. The multifaceted nature of HF demands a holistic approach that integrates medical interventions with patient education, lifestyle modifications, and meticulous monitoring.

Throughout this book, we delve into the intricacies of HF management from a nursing perspective, emphasizing evidence-based practices, therapeutic innovations, and compassionate patient care. By equipping healthcare providers with comprehensive knowledge and practical tools, we aim to enhance the standard of care and empower nurses in their crucial role in alleviating the burden of heart failure to individuals and their relatives.

Join us as we explore the dynamic landscape of HF management, driven by dedication to improving outcomes and fostering wellness through informed nursing interventions and patient-centered care.

CHAPTER 1
Clinical Manifestations

Heart failure can affect the left side, right side, or both sides of the heart, typically beginning with the left side. Symptoms and signs vary depending on which ventricle is primarily affected:

Left-Sided Heart Failure
- Dyspnea on exertion
- Crackles and tightness in the lungs.
- Initially dry, nonproductive cough
- Frothy sputum, sometimes blood-tinged
- Inadequate tissue perfusion
- Weak, thready pulse
- Tachycardia (rapid heart rate)
- Oliguria (reduced urine output), nocturia (increased urination at night)
- Fatigue

Right-Sided Heart Failure
- Congestion in viscera (organs) and peripheral tissues
- Edema (swelling) in the lower extremities
- Enlargement of the liver (hepatomegaly)

- Ascites, or fluid buildup in the abdomen
- Anorexia (loss of appetite), nausea
- Weakness
- Weight gain due to fluid retention

Heart failure was historically referred to as congestive heart failure due to vascular congestion, but terms such as chronic heart failure, cardiac decompensation, cardiac insufficiency, and ventricular failure are now more commonly used by cardiac specialists.

Nursing Care Plans & Management

Nurses significantly influence patient outcomes in heart failure by focusing on education and monitoring despite the condition's high morbidity and mortality rates. Patient education empowers individuals, improves adherence to treatment plans, and prevents complications. Diligent monitoring allows for early intervention, reducing risks and enhancing patient outcomes. Nurses play a critical role in mitigating morbidity and mortality associated with heart failure.

Priority Nursing Interventions
The following nursing priorities are crucial for managing patients with congestive heart failure:

1. Enhance Myocardial Contractility and Perfusion: Improve the heart's pumping ability to ensure adequate organ perfusion through medication administration, continuous vital signs monitoring, and optimizing fluid balance.

2. Manage Fluid Volume: Monitor fluid intake and output, assess for signs of fluid retention, administer diuretics as prescribed, monitor daily weights, and promote adherence to a low-sodium diet.

3. Prevent Complications: Monitor closely for and manage potential complications such as pulmonary edema, arrhythmias, and thromboembolism through vigilant monitoring, medication administration, and patient education.

4. Promote Activity Tolerance: Encourage patients to engage in 30 minutes of daily physical

activity as tolerated, collaborate on establishing a manageable activity schedule, and prioritize activities to improve endurance.

5. Réduce Anxiety: Provide comfort measures, offer psychological support, and teach relaxation techniques to alleviate anxiety related to the condition.

6. Empower Patients: Encourage patients to express concerns, involve them in decision-making regarding their care, and empower them to actively participate in their treatment plan.

7. Provide Disease Education and Prevention: Educate patients about heart failure, its impact on health and daily living, prognosis, necessary lifestyle modifications, the importance of medication adherence, and the signs of worsening symptoms requiring prompt medical attention.

Nursing Assessment

Nursing assessment for patients with heart failure focuses on evaluating treatment effectiveness and patient adherence to self-care strategies.

Monitoring and promptly reporting worsening signs and symptoms of heart failure are crucial for adjusting therapy. Additionally, addressing the patient's emotional well-being is essential, as heart failure is a chronic condition often associated with depression and psychosocial issues.

Health History

- Evaluate symptoms such as dyspnea, fatigue, edema, and any sleep disturbances, especially those interrupted by sudden shortness of breath.

- Assess the patient's understanding of heart failure, their strategies for self-management, and their ability and willingness to adhere to these strategies.

Physical Examination

- Auscultate lung fields for crackles and wheezes.

- Listen to the heart for the presence of an S3 heart sound.

- Check jugular venous distention (JVD) for signs of distention.

- Evaluate sensorium and level of consciousness.

- Assess dependent body parts for perfusion status and edema.
- Check for hepatojugular reflux when assessing the liver.
- Monitor urinary output closely to establish a baseline for evaluating the effectiveness of diuretic therapy.
- Weigh the patient daily to monitor fluid status, whether in the hospital or at home.

Assessment of Subjective and Objective Data

- Monitor for tachycardia (increased heart rate), ECG changes, and fluctuations in blood pressure (hypotension/hypertension).
- Pay attention to the S3, S4, and other cardiac tones.
- Note any decrease in urine output (oliguria) and assess peripheral pulses.
- Inquire about symptoms such as orthopnea, crackles, JVD, edema, chest pain, weakness, fatigue, and changes in vital signs.
- Check for dysrhythmias, dyspnea, pallor, diaphoresis, weight gain, respiratory distress, and abnormal breath sounds.

Assessment of Factors Related to Congestive Heart Failure:
- Altered blood circulation
- Changes in myocardial contractility or inotropic status
- Irregularities in heart rate, rhythm, or electrical conduction
- Decreased cardiac output
- Structural abnormalities (e.g., valvular defects, ventricular aneurysm)
- Limited cardiac reserve
- Adverse effects of medications
- Imbalance between oxygen supply and demand
- Prolonged periods of bed rest
- Immobility
- Decreased glomerular filtration rate due to reduced cardiac output or increased antidiuretic hormone (ADH) secretion, leading to sodium and water retention
- Fluctuations in glomerular filtration rate
- Use of diuretic medications
- Lack of comprehension
- Misunderstandings regarding the relationships between cardiac function, disease, and heart failure
- Invasive medical procedures

- Extended hospital stays
- Alveolar edema caused by elevated ventricular pressure
- Retention of respiratory secretions
- Heightened metabolic rate resulting from pneumonia

Nursing Diagnosis

Following a comprehensive assessment, nursing diagnoses are developed to address the specific challenges associated with heart failure, guided by the nurse's clinical judgment and understanding of the patient's health condition. While nursing diagnoses provide a framework for organizing care, their applicability may vary across clinical contexts. In practice, specific nursing diagnostic labels may not always be prominently used compared to other components of the care plan. Ultimately, it is the nurse's expertise and judgment that shape individualized care plans tailored to meet each patient's unique needs and priorities. Nevertheless, for those who find utility in nursing diagnosis labels, here are some examples to consider:

1. Decreased Cardiac Output related to impaired myocardial function as evidenced by fatigue, dyspnea, and abnormal heart rate or blood pressure.

2. Risk for Ineffective Health Maintenance related to lack of knowledge regarding diagnostic and laboratory procedures essential for monitoring heart failure status.

3. Impaired Gas Exchange as shown by orthopnea, paroxysmal nocturnal dyspnea, and hypoxemia, which are linked to fluid excess and lung congestion.

4. Overabundance of Fluid Weight gain, ascites, and peripheral edema are indicators of volume due to impaired renal perfusion and cardiac function.

5. Acute Pain related to decreased myocardial oxygenation as evidenced by reports of chest pain or discomfort exacerbated by physical exertion or stress.

6. Ineffective Tissue Perfusion (cardiopulmonary) related to decreased cardiac output as evidenced by altered mental status, cool and clammy skin, and decreased urine output.

7. Imbalanced Nutrition: Less Than Body Requirements related to dietary restrictions and fluid management in heart failure as evidenced by confusion about low-sodium diet recommendations and fluid intake limits.

8. Activity Intolerance related to imbalance between oxygen supply and demand as evidenced by fatigue, dyspnea on exertion, and decreased endurance.

9. Anxiety related to changes in health status and uncertainty about the future due to heart failure diagnosis as evidenced by verbalized worries about their condition, restlessness, frequent questions about prognosis, and concerns regarding the impact of illness on family roles and responsibilities.

Nursing Goals

Key objectives for patients with heart failure encompass promoting physical activity, reducing fatigue, managing symptoms of fluid overload, addressing anxiety, fostering patient autonomy in decision-making, and delivering comprehensive health education to both the patient and their family. Specific goals and expected outcomes may include:

1. Optimize Cardiac Output: The patient will demonstrate optimal cardiac output, evidenced by vital signs within acceptable parameters, absence or controlled dysrhythmias, and absence of heart failure symptoms.

2. Reduce Cardiac Workload: The patient will engage in activities that decrease cardiac workload.

3. Promote Self-Care: The patient will actively participate in desired activities and independently meet self-care needs.

4. Manage Fluid Volume: The patient will keep their fluid volume stable, which will be

demonstrated by edema-free, stable weight, clear or clearing breath sounds, balanced intake and output, and vital signs that are within acceptable ranges.

5. Understand Dietary Restrictions: The patient will verbalize understanding of individual dietary and fluid restrictions.

6. Maintain Skin Integrity: The patient will prioritize maintaining skin integrity.

7. Manage Pain: The patient will effectively manage pain.

8. Address Anxiety: The patient will identify strategies to reduce anxiety.

9. Improve Concentration: The patient will exhibit improved concentration.

10. Adhere to Treatment Regimen: The patient will actively participate in their treatment regimen according to their abilities and circumstances.

Nursing Interventions and Actions

Therapeutic strategies and nursing interventions for patients with congestive heart failure may involve:

1. Implementing Interventions to Address Decreased Cardiac Output
2. Monitoring Diagnostic Procedures and Laboratory Studies
3. Administering Medications and Providing Pharmacological Interventions
4. Maintaining or Enhancing Respiratory Function
5. Managing Fluid Volume and Electrolyte Imbalance
6. Providing Perioperative Nursing Care
7. Managing Acute Pain and Discomfort
8. Promoting Adequate Tissue Perfusion and Addressing Reduced Cardiac Perfusion
9. Encouraging Optimal Nutritional Balance and Ensuring Compliance with Low-Sodium Diet
10. Preserving Skin Integrity and Preventing Pressure Ulcers
11. Addressing Decreased Activity Tolerance and Managing Fatigue
12. Alleviating Anxiety, Reducing Fear, and Enhancing Coping Skills

13. Implementing Health Education and Patient Teaching

1. Initiating Interventions for Decrease in Cardiac Output

A decline in cardiac output in congestive heart failure stems from myocardial weakening or stiffening, impairing the heart's ability to contract and relax effectively. Implementing nursing interventions for decreased cardiac output in these patients is crucial to halt disease progression and mitigate complications. Timely recognition and management of reduced cardiac output can significantly enhance patient outcomes and quality of life.

1. Assess Apical Pulse and Monitor Heart Rate

Tachycardia serves as an early indicator of heart failure. Elevated heart rate represents the body's initial compensatory mechanism in response to diminished cardiac output (CO). Initially beneficial, sustained tachycardia can exacerbate heart failure over time. Effective heart rate management has been correlated with improved clinical results, including reduced hospital admissions and mortality rates.

2. Conduct a thorough health assessment, emphasizing HF symptoms and self-care approaches.

Gaining insight into the patient's medical history is essential for recognizing indications of deteriorating HF and evaluating the patient's grasp of and compliance with self-care tactics.

3. Assess Heart Sounds Continuation

During auscultation, an additional heart sound, such as S3 or ventricular gallop, may be detected (S3 mixtape here). This occurs due to a substantial influx of fluid into the ventricle during early diastole (Drazner et al., 2003). S1 and S2 may exhibit reduced intensity due to diminished cardiac pumping function. Murmurs could indicate valve incompetence. Assessing for S3 heart sounds and monitoring heart rate and rhythm are crucial in detecting increased ventricular blood volume early, indicative of HF deterioration.

Monitoring these parameters aids in identifying cardiac output abnormalities and informs appropriate treatment strategies.

4. Evaluate cardiac rhythm and document any dysrhythmias if telemetry monitoring is accessible.

Both atrial and ventricular dysrhythmias are prevalent. Myocardial stretch, fibrosis, and chamber dilation alter cardiac electrical pathways. Atrial fibrillation (AF) is frequent among HF patients, with its incidence rising alongside HF severity (Maisel et al., 2003; Yancy et al., 2007). AF predisposes to atrial thrombosis. Other common dysrhythmias associated with HF include premature atrial contractions, paroxysmal atrial tachycardia, PVCs, multifocal atrial tachycardia, ventricular tachycardia, and ventricular fibrillation.

5. Assess for sensations of palpitations or irregular heartbeats.

Palpitations may arise from dysrhythmias secondary to

chronic heart failure. Atrial fibrillation is the predominant dysrhythmia in HF and can serve as a compensatory mechanism as the failing heart attempts to compensate for reduced cardiac output with an increased heart rate (Kemp et al., 2012). Patients may report a rapid or irregular heartbeat.

6. Evaluate peripheral pulses by palpation.

Diminished cardiac output may manifest as reduced radial, popliteal, dorsalis pedis, and post-tibial pulses. Significant reduction or absence of peripheral pulses may indicate severely reduced stroke volume or the presence of severe occlusive vascular disease (Leier, 2007). Palpable pulses may be weak, irregular, or fleeting, and alternans (alternating strong and weak beats) may be observed. Assessing peripheral pulses and skin perfusion assists in determining peripheral perfusion adequacy. Reduced pulse volume and cool, pale, or cyanotic skin may suggest decreased cardiac output and inform appropriate interventions.

7. Monitor blood pressure (BP).

In acute heart failure, blood pressure may elevate due to increased systemic vascular resistance (SVR). BP serves as a guide for interventions such as vasodilators or vasopressors. In chronic heart failure, BP is a critical parameter for assessing the adequacy or need for adjustments in pharmacological therapy, including ACE inhibitors.

8. Inspect the skin for mottling.

Reduced cardiac output can lead to decreased perfusion to the extremities' skin, resulting in mottling – a bluish or grayish discoloration (Albert et al., 2010). Chronic heart failure may cause the skin to appear dusky due to increased extraction of oxygen by tissue capillaries.

9. Examine the skin for pallor or cyanosis.

Coolness or clamminess upon touch may indicate reduced perfusion. Limb hypoperfusion can result in pallor (Leier, 2007; Bolger, 2003). These findings, alongside other signs of systemic hypoperfusion, guide healthcare providers in selecting appropriate pharmacotherapy and interventions for managing the patient's condition.

10. Monitor urine output, observing changes in output volume and concentration.

Reduced renal perfusion in response to decreased cardiac output may decrease urine output. Kidneys compensate by retaining water and sodium. Patients may develop diuretic resistance, leading to decreased urinary output (De Bruyne et al., 2003). Diurnal variations include decreased urine output during the day and increased output at night (nocturia) due to enhanced renal perfusion while supine.

11. Observe changes in sensorium: lethargy, confusion, disorientation, anxiety, and depression.

Cerebral hypoperfusion from decreased cardiac output can lead to brain hypoxia, resulting in symptoms such as confusion, forgetfulness, or restlessness. Comprehensive assessment is essential to evaluate for associated conditions, including psychological disorders. Depression is prevalent among heart failure patients and is linked to poor treatment adherence, increased mortality risk, and higher hospital readmission rates.

12. Assess the patient's level of consciousness for changes indicative of decreased cerebral perfusion.

Diminished oxygen delivery to the brain due to low cardiac output in HF can lead to alterations in consciousness. Monitoring changes in the patient's level of consciousness enables early detection and appropriate intervention.

13. Inspect lower extremities for edema and assess its severity.

Edema frequently accompanies HF. Evaluating its presence and severity aids in determining fluid status and guides the administration of diuretics and fluid management strategies.

14. Evaluate the abdomen for tenderness, hepatomegaly, and signs of ascites.

Examining the abdomen provides insights into potential HF complications like hepatic congestion and ascites. Identifying these signs informs treatment decisions and interventions.

15. Assess jugular vein distention (JVD).

JVD assessment helps estimate central venous pressure and identify right ventricular failure. Abnormal JVD, defined as distention greater than 4 cm above the sternal angle, indicates elevated venous pressure and informs clinical management.

16. Monitor the results of laboratory and diagnostic tests.

Heart failure symptoms are nonspecific and can mimic other medical conditions. Diagnostic testing aims to pinpoint the underlying cause of HF and evaluate treatment response.

17. Monitor oxygen saturation and arterial blood gasses (ABGs).

Baseline oxygen saturation aids in diagnosing and assessing the severity of HF in acute settings., Additionally, it provides insights into the heart's capacity to oxygenate peripheral tissues.

18. Administer oxygen based on symptoms, oxygen saturation, and ABG results.

Supplemental oxygen enhances myocardial oxygen availability and alleviates symptoms of hypoxemia and ischemia Indications for oxygen therapy depend on the extent of pulmonary congestion and resultant hypoxia. Continuous pulse oximetry guides the titration and effectiveness of oxygen therapy.

19. Create a calming environment, encourage periods of rest and sleep, and assist with activities.

Reducing stressors and unnecessary disturbances minimizes cardiac workload and oxygen demand (Rogers et al., 2015). Physical and emotional rest allows the patient to conserve energy, adjusted to the severity of HF. Bed rest may be necessary during acute exacerbations, while ambulatory patients with mild to moderate

HF benefit from restricted activity.

20. Encourage semi-recumbent rest in bed or chair as needed, providing appropriate physical care.

Maintaining physical rest during acute or refractory HF optimizes cardiac efficiency and reduces myocardial oxygen demand

. Complete bed rest may be prescribed during symptomatic HF episodes to decrease cardiac workload effectively.

21. Create a tranquil environment: Provide explanations of therapeutic management, help the patient avoid stressful situations, and attentively address emotional expressions. Psychological rest aids in reducing emotional stress, which can induce vasoconstriction, elevate blood pressure, and increase heart rate.

22. Assist the patient in assuming a high Fowler's position.

This position facilitates better chest expansion, thereby enhancing pulmonary capacity. It reduces venous return to the heart, alleviates pulmonary congestion, and minimizes pressure on the diaphragm. Additionally, patients with heart failure often experience a chronic nonproductive cough exacerbated by recumbent positions,

23. Assess for calf tenderness, diminished pedal pulses, swelling, local redness, or pallor in extremities.

Enforced bed rest, reduced cardiac output, and venous pooling increase the risk of thrombophlebitis.

24. Elevate legs with caution, avoiding pressure under the knees or discomfort to the patient.

Elevation reduces venous return and preload, potentially lowering the risk of thrombus or embolus formation.

25. Reposition the patient every two hours.

Prolonged immobility, particularly in edematous patients, increases the risk of deconditioning and pressure ulcers. Regular repositioning helps mitigate these risks.

26. Provide bedside commode and administer stool softeners as prescribed. Encourage avoiding activities that provoke a vasovagal response (e.g., straining during defecation, breath-holding during position changes).

Using a bedside commode reduces the effort required to reach the bathroom or use a bedpan. Patients with HF may experience autonomic dysfunction, making them susceptible to decreased mean arterial blood pressure and cerebral blood flow during Valsalva maneuvers or similar activities.

27. Encourage both active and passive exercises, increasing activity gradually based on tolerance.

For acute HF, temporary bed rest may be necessary, while patients with mild to moderate HF should engage in at least 30 minutes of physical activity daily.

28. Administer medications as prescribed.

Refer to Pharmacologic Management for specific details.

29. Withhold digitalis preparations as needed and promptly notify the physician of significant changes in cardiac rate or rhythm, or signs of digitalis toxicity.

Due to its narrow therapeutic range, digoxin toxicity can occur in up to 20% of cases. Monitoring for toxic levels, slow heart rates, or low potassium levels may necessitate discontinuation of digoxin.

30. Administer IV fluids cautiously, monitoring total volume according to indications. Avoid saline solutions if possible.

Elevated left ventricular pressure in HF patients may limit tolerance to increased fluid volume (preload). Close monitoring is crucial to prevent exacerbation of cardiac workload. HF patients also retain sodium, contributing to fluid retention and increased cardiac stress.

31. Monitor closely for signs and symptoms of fluid and electrolyte imbalances.

Shifting fluid dynamics and the use of diuretics can lead to excessive diuresis and electrolyte disturbances, such as hypokalemia (Oh et al., 2015). Hypokalemia manifests with symptoms like ventricular dysrhythmias, hypotension, and generalized weakness. Conversely, hyperkalemia can result from medications like ACE inhibitors, ARBs, or spironolactone.

32. Monitor sequential electrocardiogram (ECG) and chest X-ray findings.

These assessments can reveal the underlying causes of HF. ST-segment depression and T-wave flattening may develop due to increased myocardial oxygen demand, even without coronary artery disease. Chest X-ray imaging may indicate cardiomegaly and pulmonary congestion.

33. Assess cardiac output and other functional parameters as clinically indicated.

Non-invasive techniques like thoracic electrical bioimpedance (TEB) can measure cardiac index, preload, afterload, contractility, and cardiac work. This assessment helps evaluate the effectiveness of therapeutic interventions and responses to activity.

34. Prepare for placement and maintenance of a pacemaker, if necessary.

This intervention may be required to address bradyarrhythmias unresponsive to medical therapy, which can exacerbate congestive heart failure or lead to pulmonary edema.

35. Assist with mechanical circulatory support systems, such as ventricular assist device (VAD) placement.

A battery-operated VAD positioned between the left ventricle and the descending thoracic or abdominal aorta assists in pumping blood into the systemic circulation. This device allows patients to lead nearly normal lives while awaiting recovery, transplantation, or decision-making.

36. Recognize the potential need for intra-aortic balloon pump (IABP) support and provide care. An IABP may be inserted temporarily to support a critically ill patient with potentially reversible heart failure. Continuous assessment is crucial to monitor subtle changes in the patient's condition, requiring expertise in cardiovascular physiology, IABP effects, and potential complications (Lewis et al., 2009). In end-stage HF, cardiac transplantation may be considered.

37. Withhold digitalis preparations as warranted and promptly notify the physician of significant changes in cardiac rhythm, rate, or signs of toxicity. Due to its narrow therapeutic window, digoxin toxicity can occur in up to 20% of cases. Monitoring for toxic levels, bradycardia, or hypokalemia may necessitate discontinuation.

38. Administer IV fluids judiciously, monitoring volume closely as directed. Avoid saline solutions when possible.

Elevated left ventricular pressure in HF patients may limit tolerance to increased fluid volume (preload). Careful monitoring is essential to prevent worsening of cardiac workload. Patients with HF may retain sodium, leading to fluid retention and increased cardiac stress.

39. Monitor closely for signs and symptoms of fluid and electrolyte imbalances.

Fluid shifts and diuretic use can cause excessive diuresis and electrolyte disturbances, such as hypokalemia. Symptoms may include ventricular arrhythmias, hypotension, and generalized weakness. Hyperkalemia may result from medications like ACE inhibitors, ARBs, or spironolactone.

40. Evaluate cardiac output and related parameters as clinically indicated.

Utilize non-invasive methods like thoracic electrical bioimpedance (TEB) to assess cardiac index, preload, afterload, contractility, and cardiac work. This evaluation aids in monitoring therapeutic effectiveness and response to physical activity.

CHAPTER 2
Monitor Diagnostic Procedures and Laboratory Studies

Monitoring diagnostic procedures and laboratory studies is crucial in the comprehensive care of heart failure patients. These assessments play a vital role in assessing disease severity, tracking patient progress, and guiding treatment decisions. They provide healthcare providers with essential information to tailor patient care effectively and make necessary adjustments to treatment plans.

1. Blood Urea Nitrogen (BUN) and Creatinine

Elevated levels of BUN or creatinine indicate reduced renal perfusion, which may result from heart failure or medications such as diuretics and ACE inhibitors.

2. Liver Function Studies (AST, LDH)

Liver function tests can detect abnormalities that may indicate liver congestion or dysfunction, potentially influencing medication dosing.

3. Prothrombin Time (PT) and Activated Partial Thromboplastin Time (aPTT)

These coagulation studies help identify patients at risk for abnormal clot formation and assess the effectiveness of anticoagulant therapy.

4. Atrial Natriuretic Peptide (ANP)

ANP levels rise from the right atrial cells in response to increased pressure, commonly seen in congestive heart failure.

5. Beta-type Natriuretic Peptide (BNP)

BNP, released from the cardiac ventricles in response to volume overload, increases with worsening heart failure symptoms (Cowie & Mendez, 2002).

6. Electrocardiogram (ECG)

An ECG provides insights into the underlying causes of heart failure. Changes like ST-segment depression and T-wave flattening may occur due to increased myocardial oxygen demand, even in the absence of coronary artery disease.

7. Echocardiogram

This non-invasive ultrasound test offers detailed images of the heart's structure and function, including chamber dimensions, wall thickness, contractile strength, and ejection fraction. Regular echocardiograms assess cardiac function and monitor changes over time.

8. Cardiac Stress Test

This evaluates the heart's response to physical exertion or pharmacological stress, assessing exercise capacity, detecting exercise-induced arrhythmias, and identifying coronary artery disease contributing to heart failure symptoms.

9. Complete Blood Count (CBC)

A CBC measures blood components such as red and white blood cells and platelets, identifying anemia, infection, or other issues affecting heart failure management.

10. Kidney Function Tests

Tests like serum creatinine and BUN evaluate kidney function, which is often compromised in heart failure and impacts treatment decisions and medication management.

11. Electrolyte Levels

Laboratory tests evaluate electrolyte levels, including sodium, potassium, and magnesium. Disruptions in these electrolytes can influence heart rhythm and overall cardiac function.

12. Chest X-ray

A chest X-ray can reveal cardiac enlargement and signs of pulmonary congestion, providing crucial diagnostic insights for managing heart failure.

CHAPTER 3
Administering Medication and Providing Pharmacological Interventions

Administering medication and providing pharmacological interventions are essential aspects of managing patients with heart failure. Medications are prescribed to alleviate symptoms, enhance cardiac function, prevent complications, and improve the patient's quality of life. These interventions are crucial for slowing disease progression and achieving better overall outcomes.

Diuretics

Diuretics are frontline treatments for patients exhibiting signs of fluid overload. They function by reducing blood volume, thereby lowering venous and arterial pressures, alleviating pulmonary and peripheral edema, and reducing cardiac dilation (Ellison et al., 2017; Brater, 2000). Diuretics play a pivotal role in managing fluid overload in heart failure patients. Loop diuretics, thiazide diuretics, and aldosterone antagonists act through different mechanisms in the kidney to increase urine production and eliminate excess extracellular fluid. Administering prescribed diuretics helps relieve symptoms of fluid overload and improves overall patient condition. Evidence from multiple controlled trials indicates that conventional diuretics reduce the risk of mortality and worsening heart failure compared to placebo in patients with congestive heart failure. Approximately 80 deaths per 1000 treated individuals may be prevented with diuretic therapy. Diuretics also enhance exercise tolerance by approximately 28% to 33% more than other active treatments (Faris et al., 2012).

Commonly utilized diuretics for patients with heart failure include:

- Thiazide diuretics (e.g., hydrochlorothiazide, marketed as Microzide) are oral agents that induce moderate diuresis and are prescribed for long-term management of heart failure when edema is moderate (Sica et al., 2011; De Bruyne et al., 2003). Thiazides are ineffective when glomerular filtration rate (GFR) is low and cardiac output is severely reduced. Adverse effects of thiazides include hypokalemia, thereby increasing the risk of digoxin-induced dysrhythmias.
- Loop diuretics (e.g., furosemide, known as Lasix; ethacrynic acid, marketed as Edecrin)

promote fluid loss even when GFR is low, in contrast to thiazides. Loop diuretics are preferred for patients with severe heart failure (Felker, 2012). Besides hypokalemia, loop diuretics can also cause severe hypotension due to excessive fluid volume loss. Furosemide additionally reduces alveolar congestion, thereby enhancing gas exchange.

- Potassium-sparing diuretics (e.g., spironolactone, sold as Aldactone) are prescribed to counteract potassium loss caused by thiazide and loop diuretics, thus reducing the risk of digoxin-induced dysrhythmias (Gao et al., 2007). Hyperkalemia is the primary adverse effect associated with these medications (Brater, 2000).

Nursing interventions and actions for patients receiving diuretics may include:

- Monitor and record the patient's fluid intake and output, including daily weight measurements. Regular monitoring and documentation of fluid intake and output, along with daily weight measurements, are critical for assessing the efficacy of diuretic treatment. These assessments help gauge the response to diuretics, determine the need for dosage adjustments, and identify any abnormal fluid retention or depletion. Changes in weight serve as an early indicator of fluid shifts. Tracking fluid intake and output provides valuable insights into fluid balance, aiding in the evaluation of diuretic efficacy and informing fluid management decisions.

- Regularly monitor serum potassium levels and promptly report any deviations from normal. Certain diuretics, such as loop and thiazide diuretics, enhance potassium excretion, potentially causing hypokalemia. Routine monitoring of serum potassium levels facilitates early detection of electrolyte imbalances and enables timely interventions, such as adjusting diuretic dosages or prescribing potassium supplements, to maintain optimal electrolyte levels.
- Educate the patient on the importance of adhering to a low-sodium diet and limiting fluid intake. Adopting a low-sodium diet and restricting fluid intake helps mitigate fluid overload and reduces reliance on diuretics. Patient education about dietary modifications and fluid restriction empowers individuals to actively

engage in their treatment regimen, leading to improved outcomes and alleviation of heart failure symptoms.

- Assess for signs and symptoms of orthostatic hypotension and renal impairment. Diuretic therapy can precipitate orthostatic hypotension, particularly in patients predisposed to volume depletion. Regular assessment for symptoms like dizziness, lightheadedness, or syncope upon positional changes aids in early detection of orthostatic hypotension and guides appropriate interventions. Additionally, vigilant monitoring for kidney impairment, evidenced by alterations in urine output or renal function, is crucial for prompt recognition and management.
- Frequently monitor serum creatinine and potassium levels, especially during

initiation of aldosterone antagonists (e.g., spironolactone).

Aldosterone antagonists, such as spironolactone, are potassium-sparing diuretics necessitating vigilant monitoring of serum creatinine and potassium levels. Close surveillance during initial treatment phases facilitates early identification of renal dysfunction or potassium disturbances. Timely adjustments in treatment or dosages ensure patient safety and optimize therapeutic outcomes.

- Evaluate the patient's response to diuretic therapy and assess for the onset or exacerbation of cardiorenal syndrome. Continuous assessment of the patient's response to diuretic therapy is pivotal for evaluating its efficacy in alleviating

Vasodilators, arterial dilators, and combination drugs play a crucial role in heart failure management by enhancing cardiac output, reducing circulating volume, and lowering systemic vascular resistance, thereby alleviating ventricular workload. Commonly used vasodilators include:

- Isosorbide dinitrate (ISDN) [Nitro Dur, Isordil] selectively dilates veins, effectively alleviating congestive symptoms and enhancing exercise capacity in patients with severe refractory HF (Ziaeian et al., 2017; Nyolczas et al., 2017; Cohn et al., 1991). Careful monitoring is essential due to potential adverse effects such as orthostatic hypotension and reflex tachycardia.
- Hydralazine [Apresoline] selectively dilates arterioles, thereby improving cardiac output and renal blood flow (Herman, 2017; Jacobs, 1984). It is typically used in combination with ISDN

(e.g., BiDil – a fixed-dose combination of hydralazine and ISDN).

- Nitroglycerin, administered intravenously, acts as a potent vasodilator, significantly reducing venous pressure and effectively relieving acute severe pulmonary edema (Levy et al., 2007). Adverse effects to monitor include hypotension and reflex tachycardia.
- Sodium nitroprusside [Nitropress] rapidly dilates arterioles and veins, reducing afterload and increasing cardiac output by lowering venous pressure and alleviating pulmonary and peripheral congestion. Continuous blood pressure monitoring is crucial during its administration.
- Nesiritide administration induces rapid and balanced vasodilation, leading to substantial reductions in both right and left

ventricular filling pressures, systemic vascular resistance, and increases in stroke volume and cardiac output without affecting heart rate. This treatment safely enhances overall cardiac and systemic function in patients with heart failure.

Table 3-1: ACE inhibitors and their impact on the renin-angiotensin-aldosterone system (RAAS), along with their clinical benefits and potential adverse effects:

ACE Inhibitor	Mechanism of Action	Clinical Benefits	Adverse Effects
Benazepril (Lotensin)	prevents the RAAS from converting angiotensin I to angiotensin II.	Reduces mortality, morbidity, hospitalizations, and symptoms in heart failure	Symptomatic hypotension, hyperkalemia, cough, potential renal function worsening
Captopril (Capoten)	Inhibits ACE, decreasing angiotensin II production	Improves hemodynamics, cardiac remodeling	Hypotension, hyperkalemia, cough, renal

			impairment
Lisinopril (Prinivil)	Suppresses RAAS, reducing aldosterone release	Decreases symptoms and hospitalizations	Hypotension, hyperkalemia, dry cough, renal dysfunction
Enalapril (Vasotec)	Blocks ACE, decreasing angiotensin II levels	Improves exercise tolerance, reduces symptoms	Hypotension, hyperkalemia, persistent cough, renal dysfunction
Quinapril (Accupril)	Inhibits ACE, decreasing vasoconstriction and aldosterone release	Reduces mortality and hospitalizations	Hypotension, hyperkalemia, dry cough, renal impairment
Ramipril (Altace)	Blocks ACE, reducing angiotensin II and aldosterone	Improves survival and reduces symptoms	Hypotension, hyperkalemia, cough, renal dysfunction

Notes:
- Mechanism of Action: ACE inhibitors block the conversion of angiotensin I to angiotensin II in the RAAS pathway.
- Clinical Benefits: These medications are effective in

reducing mortality, morbidity, hospitalizations, and symptoms in patients with heart failure. They also improve hemodynamics and cardiac remodeling.

- Adverse Effects: Common adverse effects include symptomatic hypotension (especially after initial dose), hyperkalemia (due to decreased aldosterone), dry cough, and potential worsening of renal function.

For patients using ACE inhibitors, further nursing interventions could be:

- Keep an eye on blood pressure and other vital signs both before and after giving ACE inhibitors.

- Regular monitoring of vital signs, particularly blood pressure, is crucial upon initiating ACE inhibitor therapy. These medications induce vasodilation, which may precipitate hypotension. Vigilant monitoring enables early detection and intervention in case of significant blood pressure fluctuations.

- Monitor serum potassium levels regularly.
- ACE inhibitors can cause hyperkalemia by inhibiting aldosterone secretion. Routine monitoring of serum potassium levels helps detect hyperkalemia early, especially in patients concurrently using diuretics that also influence potassium balance. Prompt interventions can prevent complications.

- Educate the patient on the importance of adhering to the medication regimen and attending regular follow-up appointments.
- Patient education should emphasize the significance of adhering to prescribed ACE inhibitor therapy to optimize treatment outcomes. Patients should be informed about the benefits of ACE inhibitors, potential side effects, and the necessity of regular follow-up visits to monitor medication efficacy, adjust dosages as needed, and address any concerns.

- Assess for the presence of a persistent dry cough and promptly report it to the primary care provider.

- A persistent dry cough is a common adverse effect associated with ACE inhibitors. Monitoring and assessing for this symptom are essential as it can impact the patient's quality of life and may indicate worsening ventricular function or heart failure. Timely reporting to healthcare providers ensures appropriate evaluation and management.

-Collaborate closely with the healthcare provider to adjust the ACE inhibitor dosage based on the patient's blood pressure, fluid status, renal function, and the severity of heart failure.

-The optimal dosage of ACE inhibitors must be carefully adjusted to align with the patient's individual parameters, including their blood pressure, fluid balance, renal function, and the extent of heart failure. This collaborative approach ensures that the medication is effectively managing the condition while minimizing the risk of adverse effects. Working closely with healthcare providers allows for timely adjustments in dosage, ensuring that treatment remains tailored to the patient's evolving needs and health status.

Angiotensin II receptor blockers (ARBs) [eprosartan (Teveten), irbesartan (Avapro), valsartan (Diovan)] are prescribed for patients who cannot tolerate ACE inhibitors, often due to persistent coughing that does not resolve. These medications act by blocking the binding of angiotensin II to its receptors, thereby preventing its vasoconstrictive and aldosterone-secreting effects. ARBs effectively reduce afterload, promote vasodilation, improve left ventricular ejection fraction, alleviate heart failure symptoms, enhance exercise tolerance, decrease hospitalizations, improve quality of life, and reduce mortality rates. Monitoring parameters are similar to those for ACE inhibitors.

Cardiac glycosides [Digitalis (Lanoxin)

Digoxin is a cardiac glycoside known for its positive inotropic action, which enhances myocardial contractility and increases cardiac output. It also slows atrioventricular node conduction. Despite its effectiveness in reducing hospital readmissions and alleviating symptoms in systolic heart failure, digoxin does not decrease mortality rates significantly (Alkhawam et al., 2019; Qamer et al., 2019). Digitalis is considered a second-line therapy for heart failure and was widely used historically. Monitoring renal function and serum potassium levels is crucial for patients taking digoxin to adjust dosages and prevent toxicity. Nurses should assess and document clinical signs of digoxin toxicity, such as anorexia, nausea, visual disturbances, confusion, and bradycardia. Serum digoxin levels should be checked if there are changes in renal function or symptoms of toxicity. Patient education on recognizing signs of digoxin toxicity, adherence to medication and monitoring regimens, and timely reporting of concerning symptoms is essential.

Inotropic agents [amrinone (Inocor), milrinone (Primacor), vesnarinone (Arkin-Z), dobutamine (Dobutrex)] are medications used for short-term management of heart failure that is unresponsive to other therapies such as cardiac glycosides, vasodilators, and diuretics. Administered intravenously, these agents increase myocardial contractility and induce vasodilation. Positive inotropic effects have been shown to reduce mortality rates by up to 50% and improve quality of life.

Additional nursing interventions for patients receiving inotropic agents:

Administer intravenous inotropes like milrinone (Primacor) or dobutamine (Dobutrex) to hospitalized patients with acute decompensated heart failure (HF) who do not respond adequately to standard pharmacologic treatments.

These IV inotropes are particularly beneficial for patients with severe ventricular dysfunction and acute decompensated HF, enhancing myocardial contractility and supporting cardiac output. Administering these medications helps maintain adequate perfusion in critically ill patients. Monitor blood pressure closely before and during the administration of milrinone, as it can precipitate hypotension.

Due to its vasodilatory properties, milrinone can lead to reduced preload and afterload, potentially causing hypotension, especially in hypovolemic patients. Close monitoring of blood pressure before and during administration is essential to promptly address any fluctuations and adjust medication dosages to ensure hemodynamic stability.

1. Monitor blood pressure, ECG, and cardiac rhythm closely during and after infusions of milrinone.

Vigilant monitoring of blood pressure, electrocardiogram (ECG), and cardiac rhythm throughout and post milrinone infusions is essential. Hypotension and increased ventricular dysrhythmias are significant milrinone-related risks. Regular assessment of these parameters facilitates early detection of adverse reactions and enables prompt interventions to ensure patient safety.

2. Administer dobutamine to patients with severe left ventricular dysfunction and inadequate tissue perfusion.

Dobutamine is administered intravenously to patients with significant left ventricular dysfunction and insufficient tissue perfusion. It stimulates beta-1 adrenergic receptors, enhancing cardiac contractility and renal perfusion, thereby increasing urine output. This administration improves cardiac function and supports adequate organ perfusion in critically ill patients.

3. Monitor heart rate and rhythm closely during dobutamine

administration, as it may elevate heart rate and precipitate ectopic beats and tachydysrhythmias.

Dobutamine's action in stimulating beta-1 adrenergic receptors can increase heart rate and lead to ectopic beats and tachydysrhythmias. Regular monitoring of heart rate and rhythm facilitates early detection of abnormalities or adverse effects. Timely intervention can manage dysrhythmias and maintain patient stability.

4. Monitor and document hemodynamic parameters, including cardiac function and volume status, when using IV inotropes, vasodilators, and diuretics.

Thorough monitoring and documentation of hemodynamic parameters, encompassing cardiac function and volume status, are crucial in managing patients receiving IV inotropes, vasodilators, and diuretics. These data provide critical insights into cardiac performance, fluid balance, and treatment response. They guide clinical decisions, dose adjustments, and overall patient care in intensive care settings.

5. Assess the necessity for continuous IV inotropic therapy at home if discontinuation is impractical for patients with end-stage heart failure.

In cases where discontinuation of IV inotropes proves challenging for patients with end-stage heart failure, evaluate the suitability for continuous IV inotropic therapy at home. Assessing treatment response, stability, and prognosis informs decisions regarding home-based therapy. Ongoing therapy mandates meticulous monitoring and coordination with healthcare providers to ensure safety and optimize heart failure management.

1. Monitor vital signs, including blood pressure and heart rate, before and after administering beta-blockers.

Regular monitoring of vital signs, particularly blood pressure and heart rate, is critical when initiating beta-blocker therapy. These medications lower blood pressure and can induce

bradycardia.   Consistent
monitoring allows for early
identification and intervention in
response   to   significant
fluctuations in blood pressure or
heart rate.

2. Educate the patient about the
gradual titration of beta-blocker
dosage and the expected delay in
therapeutic effects.

Patients should be informed
that beta-blockers commence at a
low dose and are progressively
adjusted over several weeks to
minimize potential side effects.
Emphasizing this dosing strategy
helps   manage   patient
expectations and encourages
adherence to the treatment plan
by explaining that therapeutic
benefits may not be immediate.

3. Assess and document the
patient's response to beta-blocker
therapy,   including   the
identification of potential side
effects.

Monitoring   the   patient's
response to beta-blocker therapy
is crucial to assess its
effectiveness and detect any
adverse   reactions.   Close
evaluation and documentation of

side effects such as dizziness, hypotension, bradycardia, fatigue, and depression are essential for healthcare providers to make informed decisions regarding appropriate interventions or adjustments in dosage.

1. Provide support and reassurance to patients experiencing side effects during the initial phase of beta-blocker treatment.

Side effects from beta-blockers are most prevalent in the early weeks of treatment. Patients may encounter symptoms like dizziness, hypotension, bradycardia, fatigue, and depression. Offering support, reassurance, and education about the transient nature of these side effects can alleviate patient concerns and improve adherence to the treatment plan.

2. Assess the patient's respiratory status, particularly in those with a history of bronchospastic diseases such as uncontrolled asthma.

Beta-blockers have the potential to induce

bronchoconstriction, which poses challenges for patients with a history of bronchospastic diseases like uncontrolled asthma. Regular assessment of respiratory status helps identify any exacerbation of symptoms or potential complications related to bronchoconstriction, facilitating prompt intervention and adjustment of the treatment regimen as necessary.

3. Document and communicate any significant changes or concerns regarding the patient's cardiovascular or respiratory status to the primary healthcare provider.

Thorough documentation and timely communication of noteworthy changes or concerns related to the patient's cardiovascular or respiratory condition are crucial for continuous monitoring and appropriate interventions. This information empowers healthcare providers to make informed decisions regarding adjustments in medication dosage, implementation of supplementary therapies, or potential modifications to the treatment plan to optimize patient outcomes.

Morphine sulfate

Morphine sulfate reduces vascular resistance and venous return, thereby decreasing myocardial workload, particularly beneficial in the presence of pulmonary congestion. Its use should be limited to patients with myocardial ischemia who do not respond to therapies that optimize myocardial oxygen supply and demand. Morphine is contraindicated in patients with untreated chest pain syndrome who have not received nitrates and beta-blockers (Conti, 2011). Additionally, morphine can alleviate anxiety and disrupt the feedback cycle of anxiety-induced catecholamine release.

Anxiolytics and sedatives

Anxiolytics and sedatives promote rest, reducing oxygen demand and myocardial workload. Patients with heart failure often experience restlessness and anxiety, exacerbated by dyspnea and difficulty maintaining adequate oxygen levels (Hinkle et al., 2017). Emotional stress stimulates the sympathetic nervous system, increasing cardiac workload. By reducing anxiety, these medications alleviate cardiac strain (De Jong et al., 2011). Moreover, patients with heart failure frequently suffer from depression, which correlates with higher morbidity and mortality rates (Joynt et al., 2014).

Anticoagulants: low-dose heparin, warfarin (Coumadin)

Anticoagulants are prescribed for patients with a history of atrial fibrillation or thromboembolic events. They are used prophylactically to prevent thrombus and embolus formation, particularly in the presence of risk factors such as venous stasis, prolonged bed rest, cardiac dysrhythmias, and prior thrombotic episodes. Regular monitoring of the patient's international normalized ratio (INR) and prothrombin time (PT) is essential to assess the efficacy and safety of anticoagulant therapy. These laboratory parameters provide insight into the patient's coagulation status and the therapeutic range of the administered anticoagulant. Monitoring facilitates adjustments in dosage to maintain the patient within the target therapeutic range, thereby minimizing the risk of bleeding or clotting complications.

Aminophylline, a bronchodilator

By widening tiny airways and having a slight diuretic effect, aminophylline improves oxygen supply and helps to relieve pulmonary congestion.

CHAPTER 4
Maintaining or Improving Respiratory Function

Maintaining or improving respiratory function is essential in caring for patients with heart failure. As heart failure progresses, fluid accumulation in the lungs can lead to respiratory symptoms and compromised breathing. Nurses play a critical role in optimizing respiratory care for these patients through vigilant monitoring, patient education, and collaboration with the healthcare team.

1. Assess respiratory parameters Evaluate respiratory rate, use of accessory muscles, signs of air hunger, lung excursion, cyanosis, and significant changes in vital signs. Monitoring these parameters provides insight into the patient's respiratory status, the severity of pulmonary congestion, and any signs of increasing respiratory distress that require immediate intervention.

2. Auscultate breath sounds: Listen for crackles and wheezes, which indicate pulmonary congestion and airway edema. Decreased breath sounds may suggest fluid overload or ventilation alterations. Crackles indicate sudden airway and alveolar edema openings, while wheezes can signal bronchospasm associated with pulmonary congestion. Identifying abnormal lung sounds helps assess heart failure severity and guides treatment decisions.

3. Monitor oxygen saturation and ABG results: Assess pulse oximetry values below 92%, decreased PaO_2, and increased $PaCO_2$, indicating worsening oxygenation.

4. Observe skin color and peripheral cyanosis: Note skin, mucous membranes, and nail bed color changes, which can indicate vasoconstriction or physiological responses to fever or chills.

5. Monitor potassium levels: Patients on diuretics are at risk of hypokalemia.

6. Educate on effective coughing and deep breathing techniques: Instruct patients to clear airways and enhance oxygen delivery.

7. Encourage frequent position changes: Help prevent atelectasis and pneumonia.

8. Position in High Fowler's position: Elevate the head of the bed up to 90° to facilitate maximal inspiration and secretion expectoration, improving ventilation.

9. Suction secretions as needed: Clear airways when secretions obstruct breathing.

10. Graph serial ABGs and pulse oximetry readings: Monitor hypoxemia severity during pulmonary edema. Note that pulse oximetry readings may overestimate oxygen saturation by up to 7% in patients with abnormal cardiac index.

11. Administer supplemental oxygen as clinically indicated.

Patients with acute decompensated heart failure (ADHF) receive high-flow oxygen via nonrebreathing masks, positive airway pressure devices, or, if necessary, endotracheal intubation and mechanical ventilation. Oxygen therapy is titrated to maintain pulse oximetry readings above 92%.

12. Administer medications as prescribed.

Refer to Pharmacologic Management.

13. Assist patients with relaxation techniques.

Teaching relaxation techniques reduces muscle tension and alleviates respiratory effort.

CHAPTER 5

Managing Fluid Volume and Electrolyte Imbalance

Monitoring the patient's fluid status includes auscultating lung sounds, tracking daily body weight, and supporting adherence to a low-sodium diet. Severe heart failure may necessitate IV diuretic therapy, while milder cases typically use oral diuretics. Note that a single diuretic dose can prompt significant fluid excretion shortly after administration. Nursing interventions focus on fluid balance monitoring, promoting fluid restriction, administering diuretics, and educating patients to optimize fluid balance and alleviate symptoms.

1. Monitor urine output, noting volume, color, and timing of diuresis.

Reduced renal perfusion can result in scanty, concentrated urine output, particularly during the day. Recumbency promotes nocturnal diuresis. Monitoring urine output assesses renal function and diuretic efficacy. Oliguria or anuria may indicate renal dysfunction requiring further assessment.

2. Track and calculate 24-hour intake and output (I&O).

Close monitoring of fluid intake is crucial for patients receiving IV fluids and medications. Collaboration with primary providers or pharmacists can determine opportunities for maximizing medication dosage within the same IV fluid volume, such as double concentration to reduce fluid load. Diuretic therapy may cause sudden fluid loss, leading to hypovolemia despite persistent edema or ascites.

3. Maintain semi-Fowler's position during acute phases.

Positioning, achieved by elevating the head of the bed or using additional pillows, supports respiratory effort in patients with breathing difficulties. These measures reduce venous return to the heart, alleviate pulmonary congestion, and minimize diaphragmatic pressure. Supporting the lower arms with pillows relieves shoulder muscle strain and fatigue caused by patient weight.

4. Establish a fluid intake schedule in case of medical restrictions, incorporating patient beverage preferences when possible. Provide frequent mouth care. Ice chips may be included in the allotted fluid intake.**

Involving patients in their therapeutic regimen can enhance their sense of control and cooperation with restrictions.

5. Weigh the patient daily. Monitor blood urea nitrogen, creatinine, and serum levels of potassium, sodium, chloride, and magnesium frequently.

Monitoring and documenting changes in edema is crucial to evaluate the effectiveness of therapy in managing fluid retention. In patients with heart failure, a weight gain of 5 pounds is approximately equivalent to 2 liters of fluid accumulation. Conversely, diuretic use can lead to excessive fluid shifts and subsequent weight loss. Collaborating with the patient allows nurses to assist in developing a fluid intake plan that adheres to prescribed restrictions while accommodating dietary preferences. This holistic approach promotes balanced fluid management and supports the patient in maintaining a healthy diet.

6. Assess for distended neck and peripheral vessels. Check dependent body areas for pitting edema and note the presence of generalized body edema (anasarca).

Venous engorgement and edema formation may indicate excessive fluid retention. Peripheral edema typically begins in the feet and ankles (or dependent areas) and progresses as heart failure worsens. Pitting edema is usually evident only after retention of at least 10 pounds of fluid. Increased vascular congestion (associated with right-sided heart failure) can eventually lead to systemic tissue edema.

7. Auscultate breath sounds, noting decreased or adventitious sounds (crackles, wheezes). Observe increased dyspnea, tachypnea, orthopnea,

paroxysmal nocturnal dyspnea, and persistent cough.

Excess fluid volume can cause pulmonary congestion, resulting in symptoms such as dyspnea, cough, and orthopnea. To manage fluid levels effectively, the patient's fluid status is monitored through lung auscultation, daily body weight measurements, and adherence to a low-sodium diet. It's important to note that symptoms of pulmonary edema linked with left-sided heart failure may have a sudden onset, while respiratory symptoms related to right-sided heart failure may develop more gradually and prove harder to alleviate.

8. Investigate reports of sudden extreme dyspnea and air hunger, the need to sit straight up, a sensation of suffocation, panic, or impending doom.

These symptoms may indicate the development of complications such as pulmonary edema or embolism, differing from orthopnea and paroxysmal nocturnal dyspnea in their rapid onset, requiring immediate intervention.

9. Administer oral diuretics in the morning.

Oral diuretics are commonly prescribed for patients with less severe heart failure symptoms. Administering them in the morning helps prevent interference with nighttime rest and reduces the likelihood of nocturia, urinary urgency, or incontinence, especially in older patients.

10. Monitor fluid status closely.

Regular monitoring of the patient's fluid status is critical. Auscultation of the lungs aids in detecting signs of pulmonary congestion, while daily body weight measurements provide insights into fluid retention. Weight gain in heart failure patients typically indicates fluid accumulation.

11. Support adherence to a low-sodium diet.

Assist patients in following a low-sodium diet by educating them on reading food labels and avoiding high-sodium foods, such as canned, processed, and convenience foods.

Limiting sodium lowers the workload on the heart and aids in the prevention of fluid retention.

12. Plan fluid intake throughout the day.

Collaborate with patients who require fluid restriction to plan their fluid intake throughout the day, considering their dietary preferences. This approach promotes adherence to prescribed fluid restrictions while ensuring adequate hydration.

13. Keep an eye on IV fluids and speak with your pharmacist or primary care physician.

If patients receive IV fluids and medications, closely monitor fluid volumes and consult with the primary provider or pharmacist to explore maximizing medication concentration in the same IV fluid volume. This approach minimizes overall fluid intake while ensuring effective medication delivery.

14. Position the patient for optimal breathing.

Assist patients in assuming positions that facilitate easier breathing, such as elevating the head of the bed, using extra pillows, or sitting in a recliner. These positions reduce venous return to the heart (preload), alleviate pulmonary congestion, and decrease pressure on the diaphragm, improving respiratory comfort.

15. Assess and prevent pressure ulcers.

Edematous areas are at increased risk of pressure ulcers due to compromised circulation. Regularly assess the patient's skin for signs of breakdown and implement preventive measures. Positioning techniques to relieve pressure and frequent changes in position help prevent pressure ulcers and maintain skin integrity.

16. Monitor blood pressure (BP) and central venous pressure (CVP).

Elevated BP and CVP may indicate fluid volume excess and suggest developing pulmonary congestion or heart failure.

17. Assess bowel sounds and gastrointestinal symptoms.

Progressive heart failure can impair intestinal function, leading to complaints such as anorexia, nausea, abdominal distension, or constipation.

18. Obtain patient history to identify fluid disturbance causes.

Determine potential causes such as increased fluid or sodium intake or compromised regulatory mechanisms contributing to fluid imbalance.

19. Monitor for signs of fluid overload, such as distended neck veins and ascites.

20. Assess urine production in relation to diuretic medication.

Evaluate urine output in response to diuretic therapy.

In heart failure management, severe cases often require IV diuretic therapy, while milder symptoms are treated with oral diuretics. Administering oral diuretics in the morning minimizes disruption to nighttime rest. Consider timing medication administration, particularly for older patients prone to urinary urgency or incontinence. A single diuretic dose can prompt significant fluid excretion shortly after ingestion. Focus on monitoring diuretic response rather than exact urine volume.

21. Evaluate the need for an indwelling urinary catheter.

Assessment focuses on managing excess fluid through diuresis.

22. Perform auscultation of breath sounds every 2 hours and postural monitoring for crackles and observe for frothy sputum production.

Increased pulmonary capillary hydrostatic pressure exceeding oncotic pressure leads to fluid movement within the alveolar septum, audible as crackles on auscultation. Frothy, pink-tinged sputum indicates the development of pulmonary edema.

23. Assess for peripheral edema presence. Avoid leg elevation if the client is experiencing dyspnea.

Reduced systemic blood pressure stimulates aldosterone release, increasing renal tubular sodium reabsorption. A low-sodium diet prevents excessive sodium retention, thereby reducing water retention. Fluid restriction may be necessary to decrease fluid intake and manage fluid volume excess.

24. Measure abdominal girth as indicated.

In progressive right-sided heart failure, fluid may accumulate in the peritoneal space, causing abdominal distension (ascites).

25. Palpate the abdomen and note any reports of right upper quadrant pain and tenderness.

Advanced heart failure leads to venous congestion, resulting in abdominal distension, liver enlargement (hepatomegaly), and discomfort. This can affect liver function and prolong drug metabolism.

26. Encourage expression of feelings about limitations.

Verbalizing feelings may reduce anxiety, which can drain energy and contribute to feelings of fatigue.

27. Weigh the patient daily and compare with previous measurements.

Body weight is a sensitive indicator of fluid balance, with increases indicating fluid volume excess. Daily weighing is crucial for evaluating fluid balance in heart failure patients. Significant weight gain may signal fluid retention, necessitating adjustments in medication, such as diuretic dosage.

*

28. Follow a low-sodium diet and/or adhere to fluid restrictions.

Satisfy thirst by providing oral care to alleviate the sensation without increasing fluid intake.

29. Encourage or provide oral care every 2 hours.

Heart failure causes venous congestion, increasing capillary pressure. When hydrostatic pressure exceeds interstitial pressure, fluid leaks from capillaries, leading to leg and sacral edema. Elevating the legs enhances venous return to the heart.

30. Change positions frequently. Elevate feet when sitting. Inspect skin surface, keep dry, and provide padding as needed.

To prevent pressure ulcers, nurses assess for skin breakdown and implement preventive measures, particularly in areas prone to edema-related risks. This includes proper positioning to alleviate pressure and regular repositioning. Nurses recognize that edema, compromised circulation, inadequate nutrition, and prolonged immobility, such as bed rest, collectively compromise skin integrity. Vigilant monitoring and proactive interventions are essential for maintaining skin health.

31. Offer frequent small meals that are easily digestible.

Reduced gastric motility can hinder digestion and nutrient absorption. Providing small, frequent meals may aid digestion and prevent abdominal discomfort.

32. Implement and educate the patient on fluid restrictions as appropriate.

This practice helps decrease extracellular volume.

33. Administer medications as prescribed.

Refer to Pharmacologic Management.

34. Maintain adherence to prescribed fluid and sodium restrictions.

This approach reduces total body water and prevents fluid reaccumulation.

35. Collaborate with a dietitian.

It may be necessary to design a diet that meets caloric needs while adhering to sodium restrictions for the patient.

36. Monitor chest radiographs.

This helps identify changes indicative of resolving pulmonary congestion.

37. Assist with the application of rotating tourniquets and/or perform phlebotomy, dialysis, or ultrafiltration as needed.

Although not commonly utilized, mechanical fluid removal rapidly decreases circulating volume, particularly effective in managing pulmonary edema unresponsive to other treatments.

CHAPTER 6
Providing Perioperative Nursing Care

Delivering perioperative nursing care for patients with heart failure demands focused attention to ensure their safety and optimize outcomes. Through these interventions, nurses play a crucial role in safely managing patients with heart failure throughout their surgical journey. Their expertise, vigilant monitoring, and collaborative approach are essential in promoting patient safety, minimizing complications, and achieving favorable surgical outcomes.

Several surgical procedures are performed for the treatment of heart failure, including:

1. Coronary Artery Bypass Graft (CABG) Surgery

CABG surgery involves creating a new blood pathway to the heart by bypassing blocked or narrowed coronary arteries. Nursing interventions for CABG surgery may include:

- Monitoring vital signs such as blood pressure, heart rate, and oxygen saturation levels.

- Assessing and managing pain with appropriate medications.

- Monitoring for signs of bleeding or infection.

- Assisting with deep breathing and coughing exercises to prevent respiratory complications.

- Providing patient education on wound care and postoperative activity restrictions.

2. Heart Valve Replacement Surgery

Heart valve replacement surgery replaces a damaged or diseased heart valve with a prosthetic valve. Nursing interventions for this procedure may include:

- Monitoring vital signs and cardiac function.

- Administering medications for pain management, infection prevention, and anticoagulation.

- Monitoring for signs of bleeding or infection.

- Assisting with deep breathing and coughing exercises to prevent respiratory complications.

- Educating the patient about medications, activity limitations, and follow-up care.

3. Angioplasty

Angioplasty is a minimally invasive procedure used to open

blocked or narrowed blood vessels, particularly those supplying the heart. Nursing interventions for angioplasty include:

- Obtaining informed consent from the patient.
- Preparing the patient physically and emotionally for the procedure, addressing any concerns.
- Assisting the healthcare team in positioning the patient.
- Monitoring vital signs throughout the procedure.
- Assisting with documentation.
- Providing post-procedure care instructions, including wound care, activity restrictions, and medication management.

These interventions ensure comprehensive care tailored to the specific needs of patients undergoing surgical treatment for heart failure, enhancing recovery and reducing postoperative complications.

4. Cardiomyoplasty

Cardiomyoplasty involves wrapping the latissimus dorsi muscle around the heart and stimulating it electrically to contract synchronously with each heartbeat. This procedure is experimental and may be considered to augment ventricular function while awaiting cardiac transplantation or when transplantation is not feasible. However, its clinical benefits in treating heart failure (HF) are uncertain (Bocchi, 2001). The significant challenge with cardiomyoplasty lies in its invasiveness and limited efficacy, typically resulting in recommendations against its routine use due to inconsistent outcomes.

5.   Transmyocardial Revascularization
Transmyocardial revascularization, utilizing CO_2 laser technology, creates multiple small channels (approximately 1 mm in diameter) in viable but underperfused cardiac muscle.

6. Prepare for Pacemaker Insertion and Maintenance, if Indicated
Preparation for pacemaker insertion is necessary to manage bradyarrhythmias that are

unresponsive to pharmacological interventions, which can exacerbate congestive heart failure and potentially lead to pulmonary edema.

7. Assist with Mechanical Circulatory Support Systems

Assistance with mechanical circulatory support systems includes placement of a ventricular assist device (VAD), which is positioned between the cardiac apex and the descending thoracic or abdominal aorta. This device receives blood from the left ventricle (LV) and ejects it into the systemic circulation, often enabling patients to resume near-normal activities while awaiting recovery, transplantation, or decision-making.

8. Management of Intra-Aortic Balloon Pump (IABP)

Some critically ill patients with potentially reversible HF may require temporary support with an intra-aortic balloon pump (IABP) (Reid et al., 2005). Care involves continuous assessment for subtle changes in the patient's condition, necessitating comprehensive understanding of cardiovascular dynamics, the therapeutic effects of IABP, and potential complications. For patients in end-stage HF, consideration of cardiac transplantation may be warranted.

7. Managing Acute Pain and Discomfort

Heart failure manifests with diverse symptoms that can cause distress and discomfort for patients. Acute pain may arise from conditions like angina (chest pain) due to reduced myocardial blood flow, musculoskeletal strain, or complications such as pleural effusion or edema. Effective management of acute pain and discomfort in heart failure patients is crucial for enhancing overall well-being, facilitating rest and recovery, and improving quality of life. Through appropriate interventions, healthcare providers, including nurses, can mitigate pain and provide comfort during acute episodes or ongoing discomfort.

1. Evaluate pain intensity using a pain rating scale, location, and triggers.
Accurate assessment aids in determining appropriate treatment strategies.
2. Monitor vital signs, particularly pulse and blood pressure, at 5-minute intervals until pain relief is achieved.
Tachycardia and elevated blood pressure often accompany angina, reflecting sympathetic nervous system activation.
3. Assess medication response every 5 minutes.
Continuous evaluation ensures medication effectiveness and guides further interventions if necessary.
4. Administer or assist with vasodilator administration as prescribed.
Nitroglycerin, a vasodilator, enhances myocardial blood flow, reduces preload, and decreases cardiac workload.
5. Implement comfort measures.
Non-pharmacological approaches to pain management are essential.
6. Create a calm environment.

Reducing environmental stimuli minimizes patient energy expenditure.

7. Elevate the head of the bed.

Improved chest expansion and oxygenation are facilitated by elevation.

8. Educate on relaxation techniques.

Teaching patients stress-reducing techniques can alleviate anginal pain triggered by emotional stress.

9. Educate on distinguishing between angina and myocardial infarction symptoms.

Understanding these differences enables timely recognition of serious chest pain necessitating emergency care.

CHAPTER 7
Promoting Adequate Tissue Perfusion and Managing Decreased Cardiac Tissue Perfusion

Encouraging Sufficient Tissue Perfusion and Handling Reduced Heart Tissue Perfusion are critical aspects of caring for patients with heart failure. Optimal tissue perfusion ensures delivery of oxygen and nutrients to the body's organs and tissues, supporting their proper function and overall health. Inadequate tissue perfusion in heart failure patients can lead to various complications and symptoms, including fatigue, dizziness, reduced exercise tolerance, organ dysfunction, and impaired healing.

In order to manage reduced cardiac tissue perfusion and to promote appropriate tissue perfusion, nurses are essential. They work together with the medical staff to create customized care plans that are suited to the unique requirements of each patient.

1. Assess pain intensity using a pain rating scale, considering location and precipitating factors to aid accurate diagnosis.

2. Monitor vital signs, especially pulse and blood pressure, every 15 minutes or more frequently if unstable. Note any reduction greater than 20 mm Hg from baseline or related symptoms like dizziness and changes in mental status, which can result from

both heart failure and its treatments.

3. Evaluate extremities for color, temperature, capillary refill, pulse presence, and amplitude. Signs of peripheral vasoconstriction, such as pallor, coolness, delayed capillary refill (>2 seconds), and diminished pulse amplitude, may indicate sympathetic nervous system compensation. Edema in the extremities can also signify fluid overload.

4. Assess cardiac and circulatory status to establish a baseline and detect changes indicative of altered cardiac output or perfusion.

5. Monitor changes in mental status, including anxiety, memory loss, confusion, depression, restlessness, lethargy, stupor, and coma, which may indicate reduced cerebral perfusion and oxygenation.

6. Assess medication response at frequent intervals (e.g., every 5 minutes) to gauge effectiveness and determine the need for further interventions.

7. Review results of cardiac markers (creatinine phosphokinase, CK-MB, total LDH, LDH-1, LDH-2, troponin, and myoglobin) as ordered by the physician. Elevated levels may suggest myocardial infarction and help rule out chest pain causes.

8. Monitor cardiac rhythms using patient monitors and 12-lead ECG results to identify abnormal tracings indicative of ischemia.

9. Administer or assist with vasodilator administration as prescribed. Nitroglycerin, for instance, enhances myocardial blood flow, reduces preload, and eases cardiac workload by limiting blood return to the heart.

10. Administer beta-blockers as prescribed to decrease myocardial oxygen consumption and prevent angina episodes.

11. Create a Calm Environment Establishing a tranquil environment minimizes patient energy demands.

12. Position the Bed for Optimal Breathing

Raising the head of the bed enhances chest expansion and oxygen levels.

13. Administer Oxygen and Monitor Saturation

Provide oxygen as prescribed and monitor saturation using pulse oximetry. Improved oxygenation boosts circulating blood oxygen levels, reducing myocardial ischemia and associated pain.

14. Educate on Relaxation Techniques

Teach the patient relaxation methods to alleviate emotional stress, a common trigger for anginal pain, without pharmacological intervention.

15. Differentiate Angina from Heart Attack Symptoms

Educate the patient on distinguishing between angina pain and symptoms indicative of a myocardial infarction. This knowledge enables prompt seeking of emergency care when necessary.

16. Reposition the Patient Regularly

To prevent pressure ulcers, change the patient's position every two hours.

17. Instruct on Small, Frequent Meals

Encourage the patient to consume small, frequent meals to mitigate heartburn and acid indigestion.

These interventions are integral to maintaining adequate tissue perfusion and managing cardiac function in patients with heart failure.

CHAPTER 8
Promoting Optimal Nutritional Balance and Adherence to Low-Sodium Diet

1. Assessing Patient's Capability for Dietary Sodium Restriction

Evaluate the patient's ability to adhere to prescribed sodium restrictions, considering individual preferences, cultural dietary patterns, and nutritional requirements when formulating the diet plan. This personalized approach ensures nutritional adequacy while promoting compliance with the low-sodium regimen.

2. Educating Patients on Low-Sodium Diet Benefits

Inform patients about the importance of adhering to a low-sodium diet, typically restricting intake to no more than 2 grams per day. This dietary approach helps alleviate fluid retention and symptoms related to peripheral and pulmonary congestion in heart failure. Empowering patients with knowledge about sodium restriction enables informed dietary choices that support fluid balance and reduce cardiac workload.

3. Monitoring and Assessing Dietary Adherence

Regularly monitor patients' adherence to the low-sodium diet and assess for any dietary indiscretions that could exacerbate heart failure symptoms. Vigilant oversight ensures effective management of heart failure and early intervention to reinforce dietary compliance, thereby preventing complications that may necessitate hospitalization.

4. Involving Family Support

Engage family members in supporting the patient's adherence to the low-sodium diet and encourage their participation in following the dietary recommendations. Family involvement fosters a supportive environment that enhances patient adherence. Studies indicate that family members adhering to the low-sodium diet themselves positively influence patient compliance, thereby improving overall outcomes.

5. Collaborating with Dietitian or Nutritionist

Partner with a dietitian or nutritionist to provide comprehensive nutritional guidance tailored to the patient's specific needs. This collaboration ensures the development of a well-balanced, low-sodium diet plan that promotes dietary compliance and supports effective management of heart failure.

6. Evaluating Patient Response to Low-Sodium Diet

Regularly assess the patient's response to the low-sodium diet, focusing on symptom resolution,

weight management, and overall improvement in heart failure status. This evaluation helps determine the effectiveness of dietary interventions and provides essential feedback for managing heart failure.
Of

CHAPTER 9
Maintaining Skin Integrity and Preventing Pressure Ulcers

Maintaining skin integrity is crucial for patients with heart failure, as physiological changes and complications can affect skin health. Preventing pressure ulcers, skin breakdown, and infections is essential for overall well-being. Nursing interventions include promoting skin hygiene, implementing pressure relief strategies, providing wound care, and educating patients and caregivers on proper skin care practices.

1. Inspecting Skin Examine skin for bony prominences, edema, areas with altered circulation, or signs of obesity or emaciation. Impaired peripheral circulation, immobility, and nutritional status

changes increase skin vulnerability.

2. Checking Shoe Fit: Ensure proper fit of shoes and slippers, adjusting as needed. Dependent edema can cause poor fit, increasing the risk of pressure and skin breakdown on the feet.

3. Gentle Massage: Perform gentle massage around reddened or blanched areas to improve blood flow and minimize tissue hypoxia. Avoid direct messages on compromised areas to prevent tissue injury.

4. Encouraging Position Changes and ROM Exercises: Facilitate frequent position changes and assist with active and passive range of motion (ROM) exercises to reduce pressure on tissues, enhance circulation, and ensure areas receive adequate blood flow.

5. Providing Frequent Skincare: Minimize skin contact with moisture and excretions to prevent damage from excessive dryness or moisture, which can accelerate skin breakdown.

6. Avoiding Intramuscular Injections: Refrain from using

the intramuscular route for medication administration, as interstitial edema and impaired circulation can hinder drug absorption and increase the risk of tissue breakdown and infection.

7. Using Pressure-Relieving Devices: Utilize alternating pressure mattresses, egg-crate mattresses, and sheepskin elbow and heel protectors to reduce pressure on the skin and potentially improve circulation.

11. Managing Decreased Tolerance to Activity and Fatigue

Effectively managing decreased tolerance to activity and fatigue in patients with congestive heart failure (CHF) is essential for enhancing their quality of life and overall well-being. Patients with comorbid conditions like arthritis and those with a long history of heart failure may find it difficult to adhere to exercise regimens, which are crucial for improving their condition. While temporary bed rest may be necessary during acute illness or hospitalization, encouraging daily physical activity is important in other situations. Exercise training can significantly benefit heart failure patients by improving functional capacity, reducing dyspnea, and enhancing quality of life.

1. Monitor Vital Signs: Check vital signs before and immediately after activity, particularly if the patient is on vasodilators, diuretics, or beta-blockers. Orthostatic hypotension can result from medication effects (vasodilation), fluid shifts (diuresis), or compromised cardiac function.

2. Document Cardiopulmonary Response: Record the patient's cardiopulmonary response to activity, noting any tachycardia, dysrhythmias, dyspnea, diaphoresis, or pallor. The inability of the compromised myocardium to increase stroke volume during activity may lead to an immediate increase in heart rate and oxygen demand, exacerbating weakness and fatigue.

3. Assess Other Fatigue Causes: Identify other causes of fatigue,

including treatments, pain, and medications. Medications such as beta-blockers, tranquilizers, and sedatives can contribute to fatigue, as can pain and stressful procedures.

4. Identify Activity Influencing Factors: Determine factors that could affect the patient's desired activity level and motivation. Age, pain, respiratory issues, impaired vision, hearing problems, and functional decline can all hinder efforts to improve activity tolerance. Fatigue can impact both the actual and perceived ability to engage in activities (Chew et al., 2019).

5. Evaluate Response to Activities: Regularly monitor and evaluate the patient's response to activities. Assess vital signs and oxygen saturation levels before, during, and after physical activity to ensure they remain within desired ranges. The heart rate should return to baseline within 3 minutes post-activity. Moderate continuous training, as recommended by the Heart Failure Association Guidelines, is safe, effective, and well-

tolerated by heart failure patients. Adjust exercise intensity, duration, and frequency based on patient response, both in the hospital and at home. For patients struggling with adherence, a referral to a cardiac rehabilitation program can provide additional support, particularly for those newly diagnosed with heart failure or needing extra guidance.

6. Managing Decreased Tolerance to Activity and Fatigue

Effectively managing decreased tolerance to activity and fatigue in patients with congestive heart failure (CHF) is essential for enhancing their quality of life and overall well-being. Patients with comorbid conditions like arthritis and those with a long history of heart failure may find it difficult to adhere to exercise regimens, which are crucial for improving their condition. While temporary bed rest may be necessary during acute illness or hospitalization, encouraging daily physical activity is important in other situations.

Exercise training can significantly benefit heart failure patients by improving functional capacity, reducing dyspnea, and enhancing quality of life.

1. Monitor Vital Signs: Check vital signs before and immediately after activity, particularly if the patient is on vasodilators, diuretics, or beta-blockers. Orthostatic hypotension can result from medication effects (vasodilation), fluid shifts (diuresis), or compromised cardiac function.

2. Document Cardiopulmonary Response: Record the patient's cardiopulmonary response to activity, noting any tachycardia, dysrhythmias, dyspnea, diaphoresis, or pallor. The inability of the compromised myocardium to increase stroke volume during activity may lead to an immediate increase in heart rate and oxygen demand, exacerbating weakness and fatigue.

3. Assess Other Fatigue Causes: Identify other causes of fatigue, including treatments, pain, and medications. Medications such as

beta-blockers, tranquilizers, and sedatives can contribute to fatigue, as can pain and stressful procedures.

4. Identify Activity Influencing Factors: Determine factors that could affect the patient's desired activity level and motivation. Age, pain, respiratory issues, impaired vision, hearing problems, and functional decline can all hinder efforts to improve activity tolerance. Fatigue can impact both the actual and perceived ability to engage in activities (Chew et al., 2019).

5. Evaluate Response to Activities: Regularly monitor and evaluate the patient's response to activities. Assess vital signs and oxygen saturation levels before, during, and after physical activity to ensure they remain within desired ranges. The heart rate should return to baseline within 3 minutes post-activity. Moderate continuous training, as recommended by the Heart Failure Association Guidelines, is safe, effective, and well-tolerated by heart failure patients. Adjust exercise intensity,

duration, and frequency based on patient response, both in the hospital and at home. For patients struggling with adherence, a referral to a cardiac rehabilitation program can provide additional support, particularly for those newly diagnosed with heart failure or needing extra guidance.

6. Use the 6-Minute Walk Test (6MWT): The 6MWT is an exercise test measuring the distance a patient walks in six minutes, providing insight into the patient's cardiopulmonary response (Enright, 2003). More information on the 6MWT can be found in https://www.somelink.com).

7. Identify and Overcome Activity Barriers: Identify and address barriers that may prevent the patient from engaging in physical activity. For example, suggesting seated activities like chopping or peeling vegetables can help conserve energy, making it easier for patients to incorporate physical activity into their daily routines.

8. Encourage Daily Physical Activity: Reduced physical activity in heart failure patients often leads to physical deconditioning and worsening symptoms. Encouraging daily physical activity can enhance exercise tolerance, functional capacity, and quality of life.

9. Develop a Personalized Exercise Plan: Work with the primary provider and patient to create a personalized exercise schedule that promotes pacing and prioritization of activities. This collaborative approach ensures that activities are balanced with periods of rest to prevent excessive energy expenditure.

10. Provide Safe Activity Guidelines: Ensure the patient understands safe physical activity guidelines. Recommendations include starting with low-impact activities, incorporating warm-up and cool-down periods, avoiding extreme weather conditions, waiting two hours after meals before exercising, and ensuring they can talk during activity.

These guidelines help prevent complications during exercise.

11. Monitor Activity Intolerance: Watch for signs of increasing activity intolerance, which may indicate cardiac decompensation rather than overactivity. Factors affecting exercise risk include age, presence of heart disease, and exercise intensity. While sudden cardiac death during exercise is rare in healthy individuals, those with cardiac disease are at greater risk (Fletcher et al., 2001).

12. Promote Adherence to Exercise Training: Encouraging adherence to exercise training is crucial for heart failure patients to benefit from it. Referral to a cardiac rehabilitation program can offer supervised exercise sessions, a structured environment, educational support, regular encouragement, and interpersonal contact, which can help patients overcome challenges related to comorbidities or the duration of heart failure.

13. Assist with Self-Care Activities and Encourage Independence

Providing assistance with activities of daily living (ADLs) ensures the patient's needs are met while minimizing cardiac workload. Encourage patient participation to promote a sense of control and reduce feelings of helplessness, within the limits of their tolerance.

14. Pace Care and Provide Adequate Rest.

Allow extra time for physical tasks, particularly for elderly patients who are more susceptible to falls and injuries due to decreased muscle strength and balance. Provide rest periods before and after exertion, such as bathing, eating, or exercising.

15. Organize Nursing Care to Include Rest Periods

Create a schedule that alternates periods of activity with rest, ensuring that personal care needs are met without causing undue myocardial stress and excessive oxygen demand. Grouping nursing activities allows the patient ample time to rest and recharge.

16. Implement a Graded Cardiac Rehabilitation Program

A graded cardiac rehabilitation program can strengthen and improve cardiac function if the dysfunction is not irreversible. Gradually increasing activity levels prevents excessive myocardial workload and oxygen consumption. This approach is particularly effective for older patients with heart failure, balancing the benefits of increased exercise with potential risks (Austin et al., 2005; Volterrani & Iellamo, 2016).

17. Adjust Daily Activities and Reduce Intensity

Modify daily activities to prevent overexertion and aggravation of symptoms. Cease activities that cause severe shortness of breath, pain, or dizziness. Educate the patient and caregivers to recognize signs of overexertion and ensure activities are performed at a safe intensity level, allowing the patient to speak comfortably during the activity.

18. Encourage Adequate Rest and Sleep

Promote a calm and quiet environment to facilitate rest and sleep, which relaxes the body and provides comfort. Implement temporary bed rest during acute exacerbations of heart failure symptoms.

19. Ensure Safety and Prevent Injury During Activity

Implement interventions to promote safety and reduce injury risks during physical activity. These include:

- Assisting the patient during ambulation if needed.
- Assessing the patient's ability to stand, move, and determine the necessary assistance or equipment.
- Providing instruction or demonstrations for unfamiliar physical activities.
- Incorporating warm-up and cool-down activities.
- Avoiding physical activities in extreme temperatures or humid conditions.
- Waiting at least two hours after meals before engaging in physical activity.

These strategies help manage the patient's physical limitations while promoting a safe and effective exercise regimen.

20. Encourage a Positive Attitude and Track Progress

Promoting a positive attitude can significantly enhance the patient's sense of well-being, motivation, and morale. For patients with heart failure striving to increase physical activity, high motivation is essential but might not be sufficient. They also need a strong sense of self-efficacy (Klompstra et al., 2018). Maintaining a positive atmosphere during the exercise regimen can reduce frustration and highlight daily or weekly progress.

CHAPTER 10
Reducing Anxiety, Fear, and Improving Coping

Patients with heart failure often experience anxiety due to psychosocial factors and physiological compensatory mechanisms, such as neurohormone activation (Chapa et al., 2014). Anxiety can arise from fears of health-related shocks, role adjustments, and concerns about performing daily activities. When anxiety is evident, nurses should focus on providing physical comfort and psychological support.

1. Assess for Restlessness and Anxiety as Indicators of Hypoxia
Restlessness and anxiety may indicate inadequate oxygenation due to pulmonary congestion in heart failure. Early detection of these signs is crucial for timely interventions to improve oxygenation.

2. Promote Physical Comfort and Provide Psychological Support
Prioritize physical comfort and psychological support for anxious patients. Creating a calming environment and ensuring patient safety can help alleviate anxiety. Comfort measures, like allowing the patient to sit in a recliner, can enhance relaxation and reduce anxiety levels.

3. Assess Physical Reactions to Anxiety
Anxiety can manifest as somatoform disorders with

physical symptoms such as pain, nausea, weakness, or dizziness, which have no apparent physical cause.

4. Administer Oxygen During Acute Anxiety Events

During acute anxiety episodes, administering oxygen can reduce the work of breathing and increase patient comfort. Proper oxygenation contributes to a sense of ease and relaxation.

5. Validate Anxiety Observations

Ask the patient directly, "Are you feeling anxious now?" to validate their feelings and understand their current state of anxiety, acknowledging the physical and psychological nature of their response.

6. Recognize and Acknowledge the Patient's Anxiety

Validating the patient's feelings communicates acceptance and helps them feel understood and supported.

7. Interact Calmly and Peacefully

A calm and peaceful interaction can help decrease anxiety, thereby reducing cardiac workload.

Familiarize Patients with Their Environment

Ensuring patients are aware of their surroundings can promote comfort and reduce anxiety. If a patient feels threatened or unable to control their environment, anxiety may escalate to panic. Reducing anxiety in this way also lessens the cardiac workload.

Administer Oxygen During Acute Stages

Oxygen therapy reduces the effort required for breathing and enhances patient comfort.

Provide Physical and Psychological Support During Anxiety

Having a family member present can provide reassurance. Additionally, pet visitation or animal-assisted therapy can be beneficial.

Use Simple Language and Brief Statements

Patients experiencing moderate to severe anxiety may only comprehend simple, clear, and brief instructions.

Teach Anxiety Control Techniques

When the patient is comfortable, educate them on ways to manage anxiety and avoid triggers. Excessive conversation, noise, and equipment can exacerbate anxiety, potentially frightening the patient and others.

Identify Anxiety Contributing Factors

Discussing anxiety-inducing situations and feelings helps the patient understand and identify factors related to their anxiety.

Determine Anxiety Triggers

Helping the patient identify what triggers their anxiety can provide insight into how to manage or reevaluate these threats.

Screen for Depression

Depression often accompanies or results from anxiety. About one-third of heart failure patients experience symptoms of both. Studies have shown significantly higher rates of depression and anxiety disorders among heart failure patients compared to the general population.

Encourage Discussion of Anxious Feelings

Allowing patients to talk about their anxiety and the situations that provoke it can help them perceive these situations more realistically and identify related factors.

Help Develop Anxiety-Reducing Skills

Teach patients techniques such as relaxation, deep breathing, positive visualization, and reassuring self-statements to provide various methods for managing anxiety.

Avoid Unnecessary Reassurance

Providing unnecessary reassurance may heighten worry and is not helpful for anxious individuals.

Eliminate Sources of Anxiety

Intervene when possible to remove anxiety triggers, as anxiety is a natural response to real or perceived threats and will diminish once the threat is removed.

Clearly Explain Activities and Procedures

Explain all activities, procedures, and relevant issues in non-medical terms using calm and slow speech. Do this in advance when possible and confirm the patient's understanding.

Educating patients before admission reduces anxiety and emotional distress, enhancing their coping skills by setting clear expectations. Uncertainty and unpredictability contribute to anxiety.

Educate About Anxiety Symptoms

Educate both the patient and their family about recognizing the symptoms of anxiety. Early identification of anxious responses allows for timely intervention.

Use Guided Imagery

Teach patients to visualize scenarios without anxiety or pain, successful experiences, conflict resolution, or positive outcomes of procedures. Guided imagery can effectively reduce anxiety.

Maintain a Relaxed and Accepting Demeanor

Communicate with a relaxed and accepting attitude, as a peaceful and non-threatening environment increases the patient's sense of stability.

Use Simple Language

Provide clear, concise, and easy-to-understand explanations regarding diagnostic procedures and treatment regimens. This is crucial for patients to comprehend instructions during periods of intense fear.

Offer Emotional Support to Patients and Their Families

A strong support system from family and significant others is crucial in reducing the patient's fear.

Allow Rest Periods for the Patient

Scheduled relaxation improves the patient's ability to cope. Nurses should pace activities, especially for older adults, to conserve energy.

Actively Listen to Patients Regularly

Active listening fosters a supportive environment and communicates care and concern.

Encourage Patients to Identify Their Strengths

Helping patients recognize their strengths aids in building their confidence and resilience.

Provide Decision-Making Opportunities

Gradually increasing the frequency and significance of decision-making opportunities enhances the patient's independence.

Help Patients Reexamine Negative Perceptions

Assisting patients in reevaluating unrealistic perceptions helps them develop a more realistic view of their situation.

Offer Encouragement and Praise for Progress

Regular encouragement and recognition of progress create a supportive environment and demonstrate care.

Differentiate Controllable and Uncontrollable Factors

Helping patients distinguish between what they can and cannot control fosters a realistic understanding of their situation.

Avoid Coercive Power

Using coercive power can increase feelings of powerlessness and lower self-esteem in patients.

Minimize Unpredictability by Preparing Patients for Procedures

Providing information in advance about tests or procedures helps patients feel more in control.

Support Planning and Timetable Creation

Setting realistic short-term goals for resuming self-care tasks fosters confidence in patients' abilities.

Ensure Home Safety Measures

Implementing safety measures in the home, such as alarm systems and safety devices in showers and bathtubs, is essential for reducing patient fear and ensuring a safe environment.

CHAPTER 11
Initiating Health Teaching and Patient Education

Managing heart failure requires complex therapeutic regimens and significant lifestyle changes for both patients and their families. Hospital readmissions are often due to noncompliance with dietary restrictions, fluid limitations, and medications, as well as inadequate care coordination and follow-up (Albert et al., 2015). Nurses play a vital role in addressing acute decompensated heart failure and developing comprehensive teaching and discharge plans to prevent readmissions and improve patient quality of life.

1. Explain Normal Heart Function and Deviations in the Patient

Educate the patient about normal heart function and how their condition deviates from it. Clarify the difference between a heart attack and heart failure. Understanding the disease process helps patients adhere to prescribed treatment plans.

2. Reinforce Treatment Rationale and Involve Support Systems

Educate the patient and their support systems about the treatment rationale, particularly for complex regimens like dobutamine infusion home therapy. Patients may alter their postdischarge regimen based on how they feel, which can worsen symptoms. Ensuring understanding of the regimen, medications, and restrictions improves symptom management and cooperation. Home IV therapy requires caregivers to manage infusion pumps, change dressings, and monitor intake/output and HF symptoms.

3. Promote a Regular Home Exercise Program and Provide Sexual Activity Guidelines

Encourage the development of a regular home exercise program to maintain muscle tone and organ function, enhancing overall well-being. Discussing sexual activity guidelines helps patients maintain a satisfying sexual relationship without overexerting themselves. Adjusting sexual habits, such as having sex in the morning when well-rested, can be beneficial.

4. Advice on Balancing Activity and Rest

Emphasize the importance of being as active as possible without becoming exhausted and taking rest breaks between activities. Overexertion can further weaken the heart, exacerbating heart failure, and necessitates adjusting the exercise program accordingly.

5. Emphasize Sodium Restriction and Label Reading

Highlight the importance of limiting sodium intake. Provide a list of high-sodium foods to avoid or limit, such as table salt, canned soups, luncheon meats, and certain dairy products. Encourage patients to read labels on food and drug packages. Consuming more than 3 grams of sodium daily can counteract the effects of diuretics.

6. Refer to a Dietitian for Personalized Dietary Counseling

Facilitate a dietitian referral to address specific dietary needs, particularly in cases of nausea, vomiting, and cardiac cachexia. Recommending six small meals daily and using liquid dietary supplements and vitamins can help prevent undesired weight loss.

7. Review Medications, Purposes, and Side Effects

Provide both oral and written instructions on medication usage, purposes, and side effects. This ensures patients understand therapeutic needs and the importance of promptly reporting side effects, reducing the risk of drug-related complications. Written materials help reinforce information, especially if anxiety impairs comprehension during initial explanations.

8. Recommend Morning Diuretic Intake

Advise patients to take diuretics early in the morning to ensure the drug's effects occur well before bedtime, minimizing sleep disturbances.

9. Teach Self-Monitoring of Pulse and Blood Pressure

Instruct patients on how to take and record their daily pulse and blood pressure, and when to contact their healthcare provider regarding parameters outside the preset range or changes in rhythm. This promotes self-monitoring of drug effects and allows for early intervention to prevent complications, such as digitalis toxicity.

10. Discuss Controlling Risk Factors and Avoiding Triggers

Educate patients on their role in managing risk factors (e.g., smoking, unhealthy diet) and avoiding factors that can precipitate or worsen heart failure (e.g., high-sodium diet, inactivity, overexertion, exposure to extreme temperatures).

Provide information on the negative impacts of smoking, excessive sodium intake, and alcohol consumption. Advise limiting alcohol to social occasions or a maximum of one drink per day unless cardiomyopathy is alcohol-induced, in which case complete abstinence is necessary.

11. Monitor Signs and Symptoms Requiring Immediate Medical Attention

Educate patients on recognizing and promptly reporting signs such as rapid weight gain, edema, shortness of breath, increased fatigue, cough, hemoptysis, and fever. Self-monitoring enhances patient responsibility in health management and aids in preventing complications like pulmonary edema and pneumonia. A weight gain exceeding 3 pounds in a week necessitates medical adjustment of diuretic therapy. Encourage daily morning weighing without clothing, post-voiding, and before eating.

12. Facilitate Open Communication and Lifestyle Adjustments

Provide opportunities for patients and significant others to ask questions, discuss concerns, and make necessary lifestyle changes. The chronic and debilitating nature of heart failure can strain coping abilities and support networks, potentially leading to depression.

13. Discuss General Health Risks and Preventive Measures

Highlight general health risks such as infections and recommend precautions like avoiding crowds and individuals with respiratory infections. Emphasize the importance of yearly influenza immunization and one-time pneumonia immunization for this vulnerable population with compromised circulation.

14. Emphasize Reporting Signs of Digitalis Toxicity

Stress the importance of promptly reporting signs of digitalis toxicity, including gastrointestinal and visual disturbances, as well as changes in pulse rate and rhythm. Early recognition and intervention by healthcare providers can mitigate the risk of toxicity and its complications.

15. Identify Community Resources and Support Options

Assist patients in identifying community resources, support groups, and potential visits from home health nurses as needed. Encourage participation in outpatient cardiac rehabilitation programs, which can provide additional support for self-monitoring and home management, particularly in cases of progressive heart failure.

16. Discuss Advance Directives and End-of-Life Care Planning

Discuss the importance of advance directives and communicating plans and wishes to family and primary care providers. Given the sudden nature of up to 50% of heart failure deaths, preparation and designation of an alternative contact person in case of cardiac arrest can ensure preferences for life-support measures are honored.

17. Assess for Coronary Artery Disease and Revascularization Considerations

Evaluate patients with underlying coronary artery disease for potential coronary artery revascularization through procedures like percutaneous coronary intervention (PCI) or coronary artery bypass surgery. Assessing eligibility and suitability for these interventions helps determine the appropriate surgical approach to improve coronary blood flow and potentially enhance ventricular function in heart failure patients.

18. Identify Candidates for Implantable Cardioverter Defibrillator (ICD)

Patients with severe left ventricular dysfunction and a high risk of life-threatening dysrhythmias may benefit from an ICD. Eligible candidates typically exhibit an ejection fraction (EF) below 35% and are classified as NYHA functional class II or III. This intervention aims to prevent sudden cardiac death and prolong survival. Collaboration with the healthcare team is essential to ensure appropriate selection and placement of the ICD device.

19. Assess for Cardiac Resynchronization Therapy (CRT) in Non-Responsive Patients

Evaluate patients who do not respond to standard cardiac therapy for potential CRT. Identification of prolonged QRS duration on the electrocardiogram (ECG), indicative of left bundle branch block, guides selection for CRT. Placement of a biventricular pacemaker, with leads in the right atrium, right ventricle, and left ventricular cardiac vein, synchronizes ventricular contractions to optimize cardiac output, mitigate mitral regurgitation, and enhance overall ventricular function.

20. Monitor Patients Undergoing Ultrafiltration for Severe Fluid Overload

For patients resistant to diuretic therapy and experiencing severe fluid overload, consider ultrafiltration as an alternative intervention. Monitoring of filtration fluid output, blood pressure, and hemoglobin levels is crucial to evaluate volume status and response to therapy. Regular assessment ensures patient safety and allows for adjustments in the ultrafiltration process as necessary.

21. Consider Referral for Cardiac Transplantation in End-Stage Heart Failure

In cases of end-stage heart failure refractory to other treatments, cardiac transplantation may offer the best chance for long-term survival. Referring eligible patients for transplantation assessment ensures access to this potentially life-saving intervention. Collaboration with healthcare teams and transplant centers facilitates thorough evaluation and appropriate candidate selection.

22. Monitor Older Male Patients on Diuretics for Bladder Distention

Older male patients undergoing diuretic therapy are susceptible to bladder distention due to urethral obstruction from an enlarged prostate gland. Regular surveillance for urinary symptoms such as increased frequency, urgency, and signs of bladder fullness is essential to detect potential complications. Nursing interventions, such as ultrasound scanning or palpation of the suprapubic area, assist in assessing bladder fullness and managing urinary issues in elderly patients with limited mobility.

23. Address Unique Symptoms and Challenges in Older Adults with Heart Failure

Elderly individuals with heart failure may exhibit atypical symptoms like weakness and drowsiness alongside typical signs such as shortness of breath. Evaluating and managing these symptoms effectively is crucial for optimal care. Moreover, older adults often experience decreased renal function, impacting the response to diuretics, and mobility limitations that exacerbate challenges related to urinary symptoms. Incorporating these considerations into nursing care strategies enhances outcomes for older patients managing heart failure.

CHAPTER 12
Evaluation of Patient Outcomes

The following outcomes are assessed:

1. Demonstrated tolerance for increased activity.
2. Maintenance of fluid balance.
3. Reduced anxiety levels.
4. Sound decision-making regarding care and treatment.
5. Adherence to prescribed self-care regimen.

Discharge and Home Care Guidelines

Nurses should provide comprehensive education and involve patients in their therapeutic regimen.

- Patient Education: Educate patients and their families on medication management, low-sodium diets, recommended activity levels, smoking cessation, and how to recognize signs and symptoms of worsening heart failure.

- Encouragement of Questions: Encourage patients and their

families to ask questions to clarify information and enhance understanding.

Discharge Goals
- Ensure cardiac output meets individual needs.
- Prevent or resolve complications.
- Achieve optimal levels of activity and functioning.
- Ensure understanding of the disease process, prognosis, and therapeutic regimen.
- Develop a plan to meet patient needs after discharge.

Documentation Guidelines
Ensure accurate and professional documentation of the following data:
- Assessment findings
- Intake and output (I&O) fluid balance
- Degree of fluid retention
- Findings from diagnostic research and laboratory testing
- Response to interventions, education, and actions implemented
- Achievement or progression towards desired outcomes

Creating a focused reference section for your book will guide readers to the sources you utilize and help them explore topics in more depth. Below is an example reference list structured for a comprehensive medical guide, assuming your content covers advanced interventional cardiology, mental health nursing, and heart failure management.

References

Interventional Cardiology:

1. Smith, S. C., & Feldman, T. E. (2018). Cardiovascular Interventions: A Companion to Braunwald's Heart Disease. Elsevier.

2. Kern, M. J., & Sorajja, P. (2020). Interventional Cardiology: Principles and Practice. McGraw-Hill Education.

3. Holmes, D. R., Jr., & Bhatt, D. L. (2016). Textbook of Interventional Cardiology. Elsevier.

4. Gorenoi, V., & Hagen, A. (2019). Interventional Cardiology: Current Concepts and Controversies. Springer.

5. Eagle, K. A., & Garson, A. (2019). Evidence-Based Cardiology. Wiley-Blackwell.

Mental Health Nursing:

1. Townsend, M. C. (2020). Psychiatric Mental Health Nursing: Concepts of Care in Evidence-Based Practice. F.A. Davis Company.

2. Varcarolis, E. M. (2020). Foundations of Psychiatric-Mental Health Nursing: A Clinical Approach. Elsevier.

3. Fortinash, K. M., & Holoday Worret, P. A. (2018). Psychiatric Mental Health Nursing. Elsevier.

4. Kneisl, C. R., & Trigoboff, E. (2018). Contemporary Psychiatric-Mental Health Nursing. Pearson.

5. Stuart, G. W. (2019). Principles and Practice of Psychiatric Nursing. Elsevier.

Heart Failure Management:

1. Yancy, C. W., & Jessup, M. (2018). Heart Failure: A Companion to Braunwald's Heart Disease. Elsevier.

2. McDonagh, T. A., & Gardner, R. S. (2020). Oxford Textbook of Heart Failure. Oxford University Press.

3. Colucci, W. S., & Braunwald, E. (2019). Heart Failure: Pathophysiology, Molecular Biology, and Clinical Management. Elsevier.
4. Gheorghiade, M., & Bonow, R. O. (2018). Chronic Heart Failure: Management Guidelines and Clinical Insights. Springer.
5. Hunt, S. A., & Mann, D. L. (2019). Heart Failure: Pathophysiology and Treatment. Springer.

Dear Reader,

Your experience matters! If you've found "Nursing Heart Failure Solutions: Practical Steps for Patient Wellness" insightful and helpful, please consider sharing your thoughts in a review. Your feedback not only helps other readers discover valuable insights but also guides us in continuously improving our resources to better serve you.

Thank you for being part of our journey in enhancing heart failure care through knowledge and compassion.

Warm regards,
Hamish Hutton

www.ingramcontent.com/pod-product-compliance
Lightning Source LLC
Chambersburg PA
CBHW071928210526
45479CB00002B/597